Home Remedies
For Losing Weight

Home Remedies
For Losing Weight

By Monica Sidoine,
S.N.H.S. Dip. Herbalism

DISCLAIMER

This book is to serve as an informational guide for use in the home. The remedies and procedures contained in this book are meant to supplement and are not intended to be a substitute for professional medical care. Please seek a qualified medical practitioner for all ailments. The author nor distributors takes no responsibility for customers choosing to treat themselves. Your use of this information is at your own risk.

ISBN - 13: 978-1533629937
ISBN - 10: 1533629935

Proof Read by Jasmine Ned Anunda

Printed By Create Space Publishing
United States of America

ACKNOWLEDGMENTS

I would like to thank all those who have contributed in one way or another to the completion of HOME REMEDIES FOR LOSING WEIGHT.

I thank God for giving me the vision, wisdom and good health to write this book. For all he has done and will continue to do in my life.

For the many prayer warriors who interceded on behalf of this project and also their moral support.

I thank my daughter Jasmine Ned Anunda for proof reading.

Thank you all.

Monica Sidoine.

PREFACE

The procedures in this Book was designed to be as simple as possible so that anyone will be able to follow them. Most of the items used are local things which you would either have at home, in your kitchen garden or can be easily purchased from the local market or health store for a very low cost.

TABLE OF CONTENTS

OVERWEIGHT

Overweight is having more body weight than is considered healthy for the person's height, build or age.

Obesity can lead to many diseases.

Persons suffering with obesity are:-
Three times more likely to suffer from heart disease.
Four times more likely to suffer from high blood pressure.
Five times more likely to develop diabetes and elevated blood cholesterol. Osteoarthritis and lower back pain. Pregnancy complications and also surgery risk.

These persons are also at a high risk to develop the following cancers: Cancer of the colon, rectum, cervix, uterus, and ovaries, prostate, pancreas, kidney, breast and liver.

Obesity is caused by:-
An excessive intake of calories than you can use up. Which comes from fat, protein, sugar, or starches, the leftovers are turned into fat.

Some common causes are:-
Having a poor diet, consuming fatty foods and not exercising enough.

TEAS

- Boil 1 teaspoon of cloves in 1 liter of water for 30 minutes.
  Drink 1 cup 4 times daily.

- Boil 4 tablespoons of papaya seeds in 1 liter of water for 15 minutes.
  Drink 1 cup 4 times daily.

- Boil 1oz of fennel in 1 liter of water for 30 minutes.
  Drink 1 cup twice a day.

- Boil 1oz of fenugreek in 1 liter of water for 30 minutes.
  Drink 1 cup three times daily.

- Steep 1oz each of dandelion leaves and peppermint leaves in 2 cups of boiling water for 15 minutes. Strain.
  Drink 1 cup twice daily.

- Steep ½oz of sage in 2 cups of boiling water for 15 minutes. Strain. Add lemon to taste.
  Drink 1 cup twice daily.

- Simmer 1oz of rose petals in 1 liter of water for 15 minutes. Strain into a glass jar. Keep it in the refrigerator.
  Drink 1 cup every morning on an empty stomach.

- Boil 1oz of ginseng root in 1 liter of water for 15 minutes. Strain.
  Drink 1 cup twice daily.

- Boil 1 garlic bulb in 1 liter of water for 10 minutes.
  Drink 1 cup three times daily.

- Boil a large head of celery both root and leaves in 3 ½ pints of water for about 15 minutes. A little lemon juice can be added.
  Drink it several times during the day.

- Blend one onion and 1 ½ glasses of lemon or carrot juice.
  Take half a glass by spoonful's three times daily.

- Stir 2 teaspoons of honey in 1 glass of water.
  Drink it half an hour before each meal.

- Mix 1 teaspoon of honey and the juice of half a lime in a glass of warm water.
  Drink it on an empty stomach in the morning.

- Combine 3 tablespoons of honey and 2 tablespoons of ginger juice.
  Take it twice daily.

- Steep 2 tablespoons of cinnamon powder in 2 cups of boiling water for 15 minutes. When it is cool add 2 tablespoons of honey to it.
  Drink 1 cup twice daily.

- Stir 1 teaspoon of apple cider vinegar in 1 cup of warm water, add 1 teaspoon of lemon juice to it.
  Drink it first thing in the morning.

- Steep 1oz of dandelion leaves in 1 liter of boiling water for 20 minutes.
  Drink 1 cup before meals.

- Steep 4 teaspoons of dried sage in 2 cups of boiling water for 15 minutes.
  Drink 1 cup twice daily.

- Steep ½oz of peppermint in 2 cups of boiling water for 15 minutes.
  Drink 1 cup twice daily.

- Boil 1oz of asparagus root in 1 liter of water for 15 minutes.
  Drink 1 cup three times daily.

- Boil the pith of 1 grapefruit in 1 liter of water for 10 minutes, steep for 5 minutes.
  Drink 1 cup three times daily.

- Boil 3oz of algae in 1 liter of water for 10 minutes.
  Drink 1 cup three times daily 15 minutes before meals.

- Boil 1oz of ginger root in 1 liter of water for 15 minutes.
  Drink 1 cup three times daily.

- Steep 1oz of hazel nut flower spikes in 1 liter of boiling water for 20 minutes. Strain.
  Drink I cup three times daily after meals.

JUICES

- Blend 1 watermelon including the seeds. Serve cold.

- Choose 1 day each week and only drink juice as the only intake for that day.

- Mix 1 teaspoon of psyllium in 1 glass of water or juice. Take it 30 minutes before your meals.

- Drink 1 glass of diluted grape juice 30 minutes before meals.

- Drink at least 8 – 10 glasses of water daily.

- Blend together 1 cup rice milk, 1 cup coconut milk, 1 cup grapefruit juice, 1 banana, 1 teaspoon molasses, 1 tablespoon barley green, 2 tablespoons yeast flakes and 2 tablespoons flaxseed.
  Drink it slowly.
  Replace one of your meals with this drink and don't take in anything else till the next meal.

- Drink a glass of beet juice three times daily.

- Drink 1 glass of pineapple juice half an hour before each meal.

- Put 2 tablespoons of charcoal in 1 liter of water.
  Take 1 cup 4 times a day 30 minutes before meals and one hour before bedtime for five days.

- Drink 1 cup of hot water half an hour before and after meals.

- Blend 1 cup parsley, ½ cup lemon juice, ½ cup grapefruit juice, ½ cup pineapple juice, 3 stalks celery and 2oz of aloe. Drink 1 cup twice daily.

- Drink 2oz of aloe twice daily.

- Drink 1 glass of soursop juice 3 times daily.

FOODS

- Eat lots of raw onions and celery.

- Eat 3 garlic cloves three times daily along with your meal.

- Go on a raw foods and juice diet for 2 weeks every other month.
  For breakfast – have fruits, crackers or bread, a shake or smoothie.

For lunch – have raw salad, crackers or bread, a shake or smoothie.
If you are having supper only have fruits.
Seeds and nuts can be included.
Drink lots of water and herbal teas between the meals.

- Make an onion broth of 3 large thinly sliced onions.
  Take it 3 times daily.

- Eat cucumbers daily as a part of your meal.

- Make a cabbage soup and have it once daily.

- Eat 2 large ripe tomatoes in the morning as a substitute for breakfast.

- Eat the soursop fruit.

- Eat 1lb of ripe cherries three times daily for three days.
  This must be the only thing eaten for the day.
  Boil 2oz of cherry stems in 1 liter of water for 10 minutes.
  Drink 1 cup three times daily.

- Put 1 teaspoon of lemon juice and 2 teaspoons flaxseed oil daily on your food.
  It will help to burn excess calories.

- Eat spirulina half an hour before meals.
  It is very nourishing, adds energy and will also reduce your appetite.

- Eat 1 whole fresh pineapple daily or eat 2 slices before each meal.

- Have fresh fruits at least 2 days a week.

- Eat grapefruits only for the day twice weekly.

- Eat oranges along with the pith only for the day twice weekly.

- Eat 1lb of grapes at each mealtime for 1 week.
  That must be the only thing eaten.
  Make sure the seeds are also chewed.

- Eat 2 apples daily.

- Have 1 tablespoon of ground flaxseed daily.

- Add fresh chickweed in your salad and use it daily.

- Steam asparagus and have it as a part of your meal.

- Eat oat bran, raw vegetables, brown rice, barley, rye, millet, buckwheat, berries and corn.

HEALTH TIPS

- Walk for at least 1 hour daily and at least 30 minutes after each meal.

- Keep a food diary.

- Set weekly goals and make sure that you stick to them.

- Saturated fats should be less than 10% of your daily calorie intake.

- Eat your fruits, salads or vegetables first before eating the other items on the plate.

- Plan your daily meals.

- Slow down the eating process.
  Chew the food slowly making sure that it reaches creamy stage before swallowing.
  It helps to increase your metabolism and you will feel fuller.

- Try to eat more things that have fiber.

- Aim to lose at least 10% of your total body weight in 6 months.

- Try to maintain the weight loss program.
  Calculate how many calories you need each day.
  Multiply your weight by 10 e.g. 170lb x 10 = 1,700
  Add 30% to the total. 1,700 + 30% (510) = 2,210 calories.
  Do not exceed this amount on a daily basis.

- Avoid crash diets.
  The weight is lost quickly but it tends to come back quickly and you might end up putting on twice the amount that was lost.

- Take enemas.

- Body brush daily.

- Get a full body massage regularly.

- Do 20 squats three times daily.

- Do 10,000 steps daily.

- Instead of using the elevator use the staircase if possible.

- Sip some water when you have already eaten and there is a craving for food later.

- Have 7-8 hours of sleep nightly and try to be in bed by 10.00 pm.

- Have the heaviest meal for the day at breakfast.

- Try to live a stress free life.

- Go on a detox.

- Put 16oz of hydrogen peroxide in the bath water.

- Cut out all flesh foods and also the byproducts.

- Have two meals daily, breakfast and lunch with 5-6 hours apart.

- Try to get at least 20 minutes of sunshine daily.

- Do not chew gum. It makes you hungry.

- Do not skip breakfast and lunch.

- Do not eat just before bedtime.

- Maintain regular bowel movements daily.

- Reduce your intake of salt.

- Reduce your intake of sugar.

- Avoid alcohol.
  It contains lots of empty carbohydrates which can be easily stored as fat.

- Avoid snacking.

- Avoid eating late at nights.

- Avoid fried or canned vegetables, quick oats, most packaged cereals, processed starch, all refined carbohydrates, and junk food.

- Avoid caffeine, nicotine and soft drinks.

- Avoid all white breads, white flour and white sugar.

- Do not go shopping when you are hungry.

- Avoid supper or eat lightly if you have to and make sure that it is at least 5 hours before bedtime.

- Do not take second rounds of servings.

- Do not overeat.

Other Book Titles by the Same Author

Can be viewed at this link:
http://www.amazon.com/author/monicasidoine

Home Remedies For Cancer

Home Remedies For Blood Pressure and Diabetes

Home Remedies For Headaches and Insomnia

Home Remedies For Sinusitis and Tonsillitis

Home Remedies For Constipation and Diarrhea

Home Remedies For Asthma and Bronchitis

Home Remedies For Dehydration and Vomiting

Home Remedies For Pneumonia and Tuberculosis

Home Remedies For Stress, Depression and Anxiety

NOTES

NOTES

NOTES

NOTES

NOTES